Reiki

Thorsons First Directions

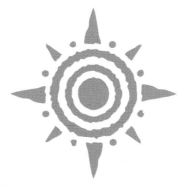

Reiki

Kajsa Krishni Boräng

Thorsons
An Imprint of HarperCollins*Publishers*
77–85 Fulham Palace Road,
Hammersmith, London W6 8JB

The Thorsons website address is:
www.thorsons.com

Published by Thorsons 2000

10 9 8 7 6 5 4 3 2 1

Text derived from *Principles of Reiki*, published by Thorsons 1997

Editor: Penny Warren
Design: Wheelhouse Creative
Photography by Henry Allen except:
PhotoDisc Europe Ltd. pp3, 5, 16, 19, 24, 31, 50, 60, 63, 70, 74, 79, 84
© Christine Boyd p23
© Horse and Rider p76
© Ametist Somanen p14, p28

A catalogue record for this book is available from the British Library.

ISBN 0 0071 0338 7

Printed and bound in Hong Kong

Always consult your doctor for any serious or long-term health problem. The information in this book is not intended to be taken as a replacement for medical advice.

Contents

Reiki

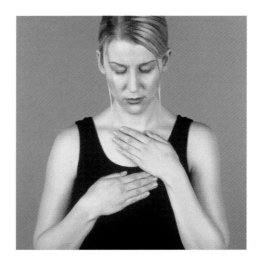

is an ancient hands-on healing system based

on channelling spiritual energy

What is Reiki?

The word 'Reiki' is a Japanese term. The first syllable, rei, means spirit, aura or subtle energy, and the second, ki, means energy, or power. Different cultures or spiritual paths have different names for this energy. In China it is called *qi*, and in India *shakti* or *prana*. In English we use terms such as life force, cosmic consciousness and divine energy. The words 'Reiki' and 'energy' are interchanged deliberately throughout this book to show the universal existence of this energy apart from any specific tradition.

Channelling Reiki

Reiki is a system for channelling life force, or subtle energy. The person giving Reiki channels energy through her body and out of her hands to the patient. It is learned through initiations in which the student is connected up as a channel by a Reiki Master.

Reiki energy is universal and has no limits. When the Reiki goes through the practitioner, she is receiving a treatment at the same time as she is giving one. The practitioner's initiation and the connection to the Reiki lineage protects her from taking on any bad or sick energy from the patient. This connection also protects the patient from any negative energy from the practitioner. The only thing that is channelled is pure healing energy – Reiki. This is why it is such a safe system.

Healing power of Reiki

Reiki is an intelligent force. The practitioner does not need to guide it with her mind, and it goes where the person needs it, not just to the area under the practitioner's hands. There is no need even for the patient to undress, since Reiki goes through clothes, blankets and even plaster casts.

After having had the initiations, you can treat people by placing your hands in a sequence of positions (*see pages* 33–41), but you can also

give a whole treatment with the hands in one position. Often I treat friends or family members while we are having a conversation just by putting my hands on their feet or shoulders. It is a kind of 'social' Reiki that brings another dimension into our relationship.

Hawayo Takata, one of the Reiki Grand Masters used to say, 'hands on Reiki on, hands off Reiki off.' The fact that it is such a simple procedure seems to be the most difficult thing to understand. People often ask me if I am concentrating or thinking anything special while I am giving a treatment, but I am not. Usually I fall into a kind of very pleasant meditative space when I connect to the Reiki.

Reiki is available to all

Reiki stands above any dogma or belief system even though Dr Mikao Usui, the man who rediscovered it, was inspired by Jesus Christ's healing miracles and found the healing formula in a Buddhist Sanskrit scripture. It is not even necessary to believe in Reiki for it to work. My sister Kerstin is a professional sceptic. Once when she had a headache I offered to treat it with Reiki. Though she did not believe that Reiki could possibly change anything, she agreed. After her first session, Kerstin had a shoulder ache instead of a headache. She was puzzled. I told her that the headache was caused by tension in her shoulders. The second Reiki treatment released her shoulders and the pain disappeared. But even after I taught Kerstin Reiki, she could not accept that just putting her hands on someone could help them. When a friend had a headache, she offered to give her some Reiki, saying that it probably would not work. Her friend's headache disappeared, and my sister is still in shock.

Reiki is love

For me, the essence of Reiki is love. As soon as I put my hands on someone, my heart opens up and I feel connected to the patient on a level far beyond personality. A pleasant energy, warm and tingling, spreads in my body and goes from my hands into the patient's body. I can feel how tension melts away under my hands. I always feel better after I have given a treatment because of my connection to the Reiki energy. Even when I treat people whom I might find difficult on a personal level, I only feel compassion. Love has no discrimination. Love has no judgement. Love is.

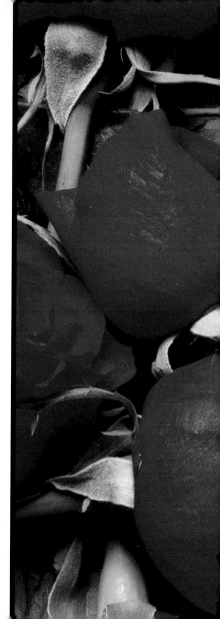

How Did it All Start?

Reiki is a method of healing that dates back about 2500 years, but was forgotten for a very long time. In the nineteenth century the system was rediscovered by Dr Mikao Usui, who passed on this 'living knowledge' in an oral tradition from teacher to teacher. These main teachers are usually referred to as Grand Masters. They form the lineage through which Reiki has been handed down and they hold the energy of this tradition

Dr Mikao Usui's story

Dr Mikao Usui was a Christian headmaster and minister at Doshisha University in Kyoto, Japan, towards the end of the nineteenth century. One morning, some of his students asked if he thought that the stories in the Bible about Jesus's healing miracles were literally true. Usui answered that he did believe Jesus performed miracles and healed

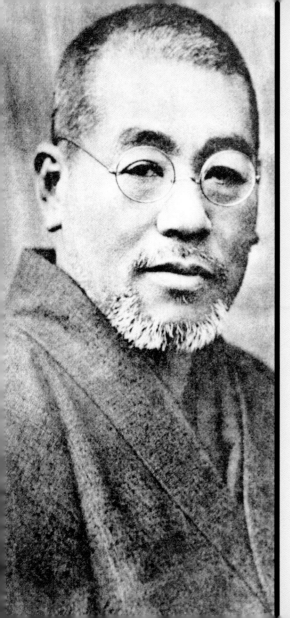

people. The students wanted Usui to demonstrate how Jesus did his healing, something Usui had to admit he could not do.

Usui took their demands seriously. He left his post at the university and went to the United States to study theology at the University of Chicago for seven years. Despite studying the Bible and other Christian scriptures, nowhere could he find what he was looking for: a formula for Jesus's healing miracles.

Knowing that Buddha also healed the sick, Usui started to study Buddhism and returned to Kyoto in Japan, where he found a Zen abbot who was interested in his quest, and invited him to stay and study in his monastery outside Kyoto. Dr Usui started to study the

Buddhist scriptures, the sutras, in Japanese. Since Buddhism came to Japan through China, he learned Chinese in order to have more scriptures available to him. Later Dr Usui also learned Sanskrit, the sacred and ancient language of India, where Buddha was born. Only then did he come across a healing formula that indicated how Buddha did his healing. Dr Usui had finally found what he was looking for. However, since he did not yet know how to use the formula, he did not yet have the power to heal.

Dr Usui's experience on the mountain

Dr Usui decided to meditate, chant and fast for 21 days on the sacred mountain, Kurayama, 17 miles outside Kyoto. This would help him unlock the power of the healing formula from the Buddhist sutras. To keep time, he put 21 stones in front of him. As each day passed, he threw away one stone.

Before dawn on the last morning, Dr Usui saw a flickering light on the horizon. As it started to move closer, he became quite frightened, but courageously decided to face it. This was the moment he had been waiting for. The light turned into a bright white beam that hit him between the eyes. It was so powerful that Dr Usui fell down, unconscious.

When Dr Usui regained consciousness, he looked up at the sky and saw bubbles of all the colours of the rainbow dancing in front of his eyes. Then the sky turned into a bright white screen. On that screen, Usui saw symbols and what he had found in the Sanskrit scriptures written in golden letters. As they vibrated in front of him, their use and meaning were transmitted to him and they seemed to say 'Remember, remember, remember!'

The four miracles of Reiki

When Dr Usui came out of his experience, he was filled with light and energy, even though he had fasted for three weeks. That was the first sign for Dr Usui that he had received a very special gift on the mountain.

In his enthusiasm, he rushed down the mountainside, stumbled and stubbed his toe, which started bleeding. Automatically, he put his hand over the toe. The bleeding stopped and the pain went away. Later he ordered breakfast in a café, where he healed a girl suffering from toothache. These were two more miracles.

The fourth miracle for Dr Usui was the fact that he could digest his breakfast without getting indigestion after having fasted for 21 days!

Dr Usui's healing work

Returning to the monastery, Usui found the abbot in bed with arthritis, hugging his blanket to his chest. As Dr Usui told him about his experiences, he put his hand on the abbot to relieve the pain. Both the abbot and Usui felt that as this healing power was a gift from God, it should be given to the people who needed it the most.

Therefore, the next morning Dr Usui started treating beggars in a large slum in Kyoto. Once they were healed, Dr Usui told them to go to the abbot in his old monastery to ask for a job and a new name so that they would find a new sense of identity and change their ways.

After many years of work in the slums, Dr Usui started to recognize people whom he had treated a long time ago. When he asked them why they were back, they told him that it was much easier to carry on begging than to work. Dr Usui learned important lessons from this experience. First he said, 'No more Reiki for free!' There was no appreciation and gratitude from the beggars. They were not ready to change and take responsibility for their lives.

Secondly, Dr Usui added his spiritual precepts to the Reiki tradition:

Just for today do not anger.
Just for today do not worry.
Honour your parents, teachers and elders.
Earn your living honestly.
Show gratitude to all living things.

Dr Churjiro Hayashi

Dr Usui met Churjiro Hayashi when he left the slums of Kyoto and went on a pilgrimage all over Japan. Usui used to carry a torch in broad daylight to make people curious. If people asked why he would say he was looking for people 'who needed light.' Then he would give lectures about Reiki in the temples.

When Hayashi met Dr Usui, he was a 45-year-old retired naval officer. Dr Usui encouraged him to accompany him on his pilgrimage of healing and teaching around Japan. In this way, Hayashi became Usui's main disciple and, after Usui's death, his successor and the new Grand Master.

Hayashi created a small Reiki clinic in Tokyo, which had only eight beds. The Reiki practitioners were all men who wore traditional kimonos while treating their patients. The clinic was open in the morning, and in the afternoon practitioners made home visits to people who were too ill to come to the clinic. Patients were also treated with herbs.

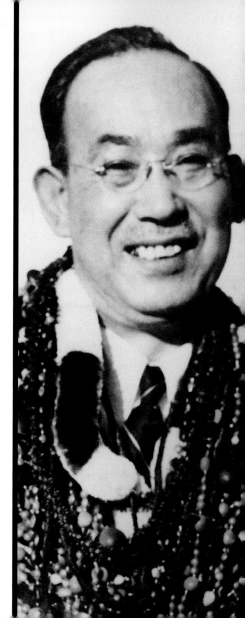

As the Second World War began in Europe, Hayashi could sense the coming conflict between Japan and the United States. He did not want to be drawn in, since he had now given his life to healing and saving lives. So he invited his family and Reiki Masters to a tea ceremony in which he voluntarily died by withdrawing his life force after having declared Hawayo Takata as his successor.

Hawayo Takata's story

Hawayo Takata, a Japanese-American woman, was born in 1900 on one of the Hawaiian islands. When she was in her thirties her husband died, leaving her to bring up two small daughters. Overwork brought on many physical problems, including gallstones, asthma, and a tumour. On the verge of a breakdown, Takata prayed for guidance, and an inner voice told her that she must first take care of her health.

Following this advice, Hawayo Takata went for surgery to a hospital in Tokyo. On the day of the

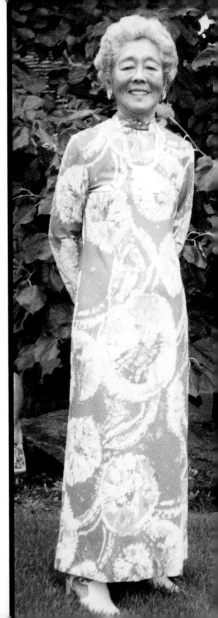

operation, when she was actually on the operating table, she heard an inner voice saying, 'The operation is not necessary.' Takata jumped off the operating table, creating quite a stir. She asked the doctor if there was an alternative to the operation. He told her that alternative treatment could take a long time, from months to a year. To show her eagerness, Takata said she would gladly stay for two years. Then the doctor took her to talk to his sister, the dietician at the hospital, who had been treated with Reiki while suffering from dysentery.

Takata's first encounter with Reiki

The next day Takata was brought to Hayashi's nearby Reiki clinic. Takata thought that the heat from the Reiki practitioners' hands meant they were connected to some electrical wires. Hayashi explained to Takata that the energy she felt was not electrical energy. It was Reiki – universal life energy. He said, 'This energy comes through me to you. These,' he held up his hands, 'are the electrodes. That force begins to revitalize and restore the balance of your entire system.'

Takata received treatments every day and was well in four months. She was so impressed that she wanted to learn the Reiki system, but was not allowed to, being a foreigner. Reiki was a guarded Japanese tradition. She pleaded her case – what would she do if she fell ill again in Hawaii? Hayashi gave in. He told Takata that, if she was willing to stay for a year and work with him in the clinic, he would initiate her into the first degree of Reiki. Takata agreed and moved in to live with the Hayashi family.

Takata brings Reiki to the West

After a year of work in the clinic, Takata received her second degree Reiki initiation and returned to the United States. Back in Hawaii, she started treating family and friends. In 1937, Hayashi and his daughter came for a six-month visit to help Takata establish Reiki in Hawaii. In February 1938, Hayashi initiated Takata as a Reiki Master before returning to Japan.

Takata taught Reiki throughout the United States and Canada for over 40 years, but only in 1975 did she start to initiate Reiki Masters. Before she died in December 1980, she had initiated 22 Reiki Masters, one of whom was Wanja Twan, my Reiki Master. The process that she helped to set in motion has created an explosion of Reiki around the world.

As Takata used to say, 'With Reiki comes Health, Happiness, Prosperity, and a Long Life.' Before Takata passed on, she also made it clear that she wanted her granddaughter, Phyllis Lei Furumoto, to continue as the head of the lineage.

Phyllis, Takata and Wanja ▶

What can Reiki do for Me?

There is not a single situation in life in which you cannot bring in the connection of Reiki. Its healing energy works on all levels – spiritual, mental, emotional, and physical.

The effect of Reiki

An individual's experience during a treatment depends on what he needs at that moment and how sensitive he is to subtle energy. Some people may just feel a general relaxed state of well-being, while others have strong physical and emotional reactions, indicating that the body's healing processes are working. Reiki is very good at detecting weaknesses in the body. It works like a flood of energy, moving blocks, increasing the circulation on both a subtle and physical level, and balancing the system. On a physical level, Reiki clears toxic waste accumulated in the body, while emotionally it allows hidden feelings of vulnerability, irritability, and sadness to surface. This is what is usually called a 'healing crisis' and is part of the purification process that will leave the person lighter and more balanced.

Reiki as meditation

Many people like to have Reiki treatment even if they do not have any particular health problem. Their experiences might be akin to meditation because Reiki is a spiritual force. I had one patient who came to me because he wanted Reiki to help him connect to his inner being. On this level, the experience might be an altered state of consciousness, seeing bright colours, or light, feeling an openness of heart, having visions and even hearing mantras.

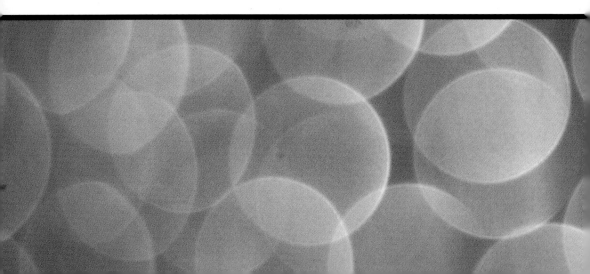

Treating ailments

All emotional problems generally respond very quickly to Reiki. Physical conditions linked to stress and tension including headaches, cramps, sleeping problems, and high blood pressure, also respond well because of Reiki's profound centring and balancing effect. As a matter of fact, most of my early clients had emotional problems or bad backs. I found that a back that had 'gone out' or into spasm would usually be relieved within three treatments.

Reiki can also have good results with acute problems. It can speed up the healing of broken bones and relieve acute pain. The mother of one of my students was in hospital waiting for surgery because her intestines were cramped into a knot. Her daughter had just learned Reiki and went to visit. She discreetly put her hands on her mother's stomach for some time. The doctors were amazed to see that the problem the mother came in with had disappeared. She went home without having the operation.

Overcoming addiction

Changes on a mental level are more subtle and generally seem to happen over a longer period after the initiations. Eva, a friend of mine, wanted to learn Reiki in order to quit smoking. I told her that I could not guarantee anything, but if she really wanted to stop smoking, Reiki would certainly help her. So much was happening for Eva during the Reiki workshop that we both forgot about the smoking. Later, when I remembered, I asked her about her smoking habit. Eva said that she had cut down her daily consumption to half without thinking about it. Reiki helps to balance the whole system. As we open up to Reiki we get more sensitive and more in touch with what we do to ourselves. We can sense how unnatural it is to overload our systems with alcohol, drugs and too much or the wrong kind of food. Reiki also fills the spiritual emptiness or disconnection that often is at the core of the addiction.

Reiki for children

Children usually love Reiki and respond quite quickly. If their parents have been initiated into Reiki it becomes very natural for children to ask for treatment when they feel unwell, for example if they have a headache or a stomach upset. Treatments are usually informal and shorter than adult treatments because children get restless if they lie still for a long time. They also tend to become quite hot during Reiki. A good way to give Reiki to a child is to do a spot treatment on the aching part. Another good idea is to have the child on your lap reading a story and put one hand on their stomach.

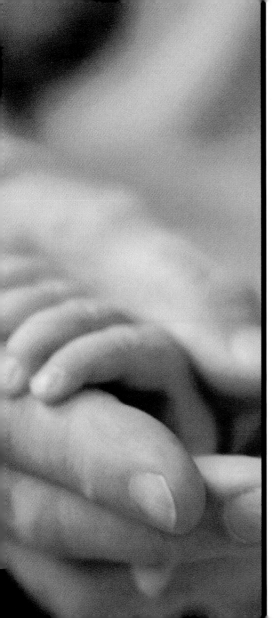

Reiki in pregnancy

It is great to give pregnant women Reiki to relieve the tension they get carrying around so much extra weight. The baby in the womb also benefits enormously. One of my editors, Diana, treated her sister who was having some pain and tiredness late in her pregnancy. As soon as she put her hands on her sister's leg, they both felt the baby moving around inside the womb. I have initiated many pregnant women into Reiki so that they are able to communicate with their unborn child in a unique way.

Dying with the support of Reiki

Since Reiki is a spiritual energy, it can help people reconnect to their spiritual selves, and help them to accept their transition. It can also help to ease the pain and fear of dying. In Lyon, France, where I used to go regularly, I taught Reiki to a nurse, Isabelle. Through word of mouth, other nurses heard about it and many of them came for initiations. Now in the hospital where they work, the nurses have permission to use Reiki for dying patients, who frequently ask for a nurse who knows Reiki to sit with them.

Is Reiki safe?

There is really no contraindication for treating with Reiki as long as the patient is willing to take responsibility for his or her reactions. Nobody can promise that a healing will occur. Only by trying can you see how a person responds.

Benefits of Reiki

As the life energy flows into the patient, it brings about a wide range of healing effects including:

Physical effects

Reduces muscular tension

Lifts headaches

Soothes stomach aches

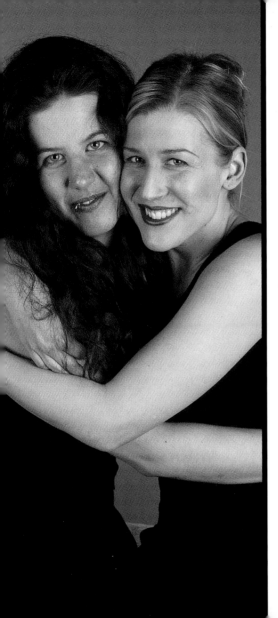

Eases pain
Balances energies
Clears toxins
Relieves fatigue
Increases energy
Promotes refreshing sleep
Strengthens natural self-healing
mechanisms

Emotional and mental effects

Promotes calm and well-being
Relaxes body and mind
Aids meditation
Relieves stress
Enhances creativity
Encourages emotional release
Soothes emotional distress
Helps unlock suppressed feelings
Promotes a peaceful, positive outlook

Visiting a Practitioner

How to find a reputable practitioner or Reiki Master

As Reiki has spread throughout the world, treatment is now offered in nearly every complementary health centre. There are three levels of Reiki. The first degree is hands-on healing. Second degree is being able to send distant healing. The third degree, or Master level, allows you to teach Reiki to others.

For you to receive a treatment, the practitioner just needs to be on the first or second level, but she can also be a Master. But if you want to learn Reiki, you have to go to a Master. The first and second degree levels can be taught in two two-day Reiki workshops, while becoming a Reiki Master is a long-term project. The Reiki Alliance (*see page* 89) was formed to act as a support group for people who are already Masters and to give guidelines for this delicate process. It will only accept members who follow professional standards, such as a code of ethics. A list of hundreds of Reiki Masters worldwide is published annually by the Reiki Alliance.

There is also a Reiki Association in the UK (*see page* 89) which has two lists, one with vetted practitioners and one list of Reiki Masters showing their particular lineage.

Word-of-mouth recommendations

The traditional way to find a Reiki Master or practitioner is through word of mouth. Takata was against advertising; she felt the Reiki itself should attract people. I have always liked this concept. Someone has a powerful experience with Reiki and tells someone else, who tells another person. I have seen many examples of

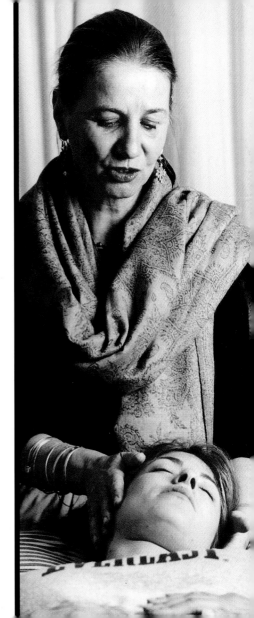

a whole group of people drawn to Reiki's healing power. I once met a recovered alcoholic who spent most of his days in a café in Northern Paris. After I initiated him into Reiki, he talked about it to the people working in the café and to the customers. In a short time I had initiated the waiter, the waiter's sister, mother, and girlfriend, the café owner, his wife, and brother-in-law, who wanted to do Reiki on his 300 sheep!

What to expect when you get there

Reiki is normally given as hands-on treatment. You will be asked to take your shoes off and lie down on your back on a massage table or on a futon on the floor. I prefer working on the floor since I feel more at ease there. You do not need to undress, as the energy can penetrate clothes. Usually I keep a blanket nearby in case the patient feels cold. I have noticed a release

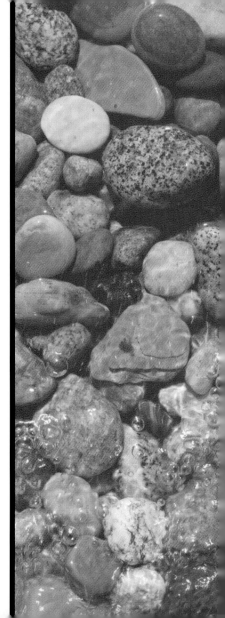

of emotion is often preceded by a sensation of cold. Also, being covered by a blanket can help people feel safe.

I sit next to the patient, with a straight spine, and start the treatment on the head, putting my hands over the eyes and forehead. The Reiki immediately connects without any ceremonies or intentions on my part, and my hands tingle as they start to get warmer. I do not apply any pressure or hold them away from the body of the client. In fact I do nothing at all! I just let the energy coming through me do the work. I can, myself, feel the pleasant flow of Reiki going though me into the patient as I am settling into the session. When the heat of my hands subsides I move to the next hand position. I move the position of my hands each time I sense a stillness, and very quickly my hands seem to find their own rhythm.

I continue the treatment down the front of the body and then ask the client to turn over so I can treat the back, from the shoulders all the way down to the sacrum. I end the treatment with an energy stroke down the spine to bring the patient's attention back to her body. At the end of the session the patient is usually extremely relaxed; some people almost fall asleep. I always give the person some time to come to, so as not to jolt her new, balanced state.

If a person has a lot of emotional release during a treatment, I tend to keep my hands on the head or heart position throughout. It feels more as though I am there with her, in case she wants to talk about what she is experiencing. However, I try to avoid giving advice or calming people down. I let the energy do the work and remain as a supportive witness. It is a personal choice if the client wants to talk or not. It does not affect the healing process, which happens on a much deeper level.

Length and frequency of treatments

A Reiki treatment usually lasts between an hour and one-and-a-half hours. The energy keeps moving in the body after the treatment for about 24 hours, so it is common practice to give three to four treatments on consecutive days.

Having Reiki is starting a process. Every session is different; with each session the energy reaches deeper into the person. It is a good idea to have three sessions to start with. Some people may have very strong reactions during or after the first session. The second session, however, will smooth this over and the practitioner will explain the benefits of the 'clear-out'. During the third treatment people usually feel quite good. Depending on your particular problem, you can then decide to have a treatment once or twice a week. There is no set pattern or number of treatments. To some extent, the number of sessions required depends on the problem: the more serious it is, the more Reiki is needed.

How do I do It?

How to give hands-on Reiki

There are two methods of healing with Reiki: first degree is hands-on healing; second degree is distant healing. To learn how to give a Reiki first-degree treatment, you need to be 'initiated', which means attending a workshop. These are taught in four two-hour sessions. The format is still pretty much the same as in Takata's day, except that she did the four sessions over four separate days. The group is normally quite small, usually no more than 12 people. No previous knowledge is required. Many people who decide to be initiated have had experiences of Reiki treatments, but this is not necessary.

As Reiki is an oral tradition, I start by telling the story of how I came to learn Reiki. While I am telling my story, I touch on many things that the students will go through or feel themselves. I also talk about subtle energy in general and try to convey the experience of Reiki. But Reiki is not something that can be 'learned' from a book. Takata would not allow anyone to take notes during these talks. The initiations open up your intuition and inner knowing: you become the book yourself. I tell the students about my teacher, Wanja, and the stories about the Grand Masters, Usui, Hayashi, and Takata. Then, if there are no questions, it is time for the first initiation.

The initiation

Without being initiated, it is not possible to channel Reiki. The initiation 'links up' the student as a Reiki channel. It is done with touch and silent mantras from the Reiki Master, while the students have their eyes closed and their hands folded in a praying position. There are four initiations for the first degree of Reiki. Each takes only a couple of minutes and each one opens up the student on a deeper level. The last initiation closes the initiation process. Usually, one initiation will be experienced as stronger than the others.

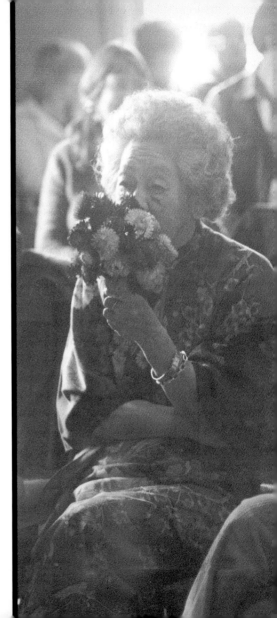

The first degree initiations open up the subtle energy centres (called *chakras* in some traditions) of the students' heart, hands, and top of the head so they can channel healing energies through their hands. The first two initiations are given on the first day and the next two on the second day. It is important to have time between initiations so students can 'digest the energy'. The initiations can give rise to a lot of powerful inner changes and transformations. The timing of the initiations might vary according to the situation, but normally not more than two initiations should be given on one day. That would create too much heat in the body. It is also important that the students do not take drugs or drink alcohol during the workshop since the system is quite open and sensitive.

When giving Reiki workshops, I have a small room that is set aside for initiations. I put pictures of the Grand Masters, a candle, and a flower on a table as a focus. I love to look at their smiling faces and the peace they emit. But if students think that this is a kind of mystical ceremony, I can do the initiation just as well without any pictures. I only need a chair for the student to sit on. I initiate the students one at a time. Takata sometimes used to initiate a few students at a time but I prefer to have a private moment with each student. Some students have strong emotional or spiritual experiences of the initiations. Others might want to say something in confidence.

What is the initiation like?

The strongest spiritual experience people usually have comes during the initiations, because that is when the link-up to a higher power takes place. This is an experience that is hard to put into words. There can be a sense of connecting to the divine energy, and a sense of this energy streaming down into the student. Some people see light or brilliant colours. One of my students had a vision of her spiritual teacher. People experience a feeling of the heart opening – it can be a very emotional moment. There often is a sense of feeling high or 'blissed out'. I had one student who could not stop laughing. He kept laughing all night long after the first initiations and felt high with a sense of extreme well-being for about two weeks after the workshop. Another woman, a friend of mine, who also felt this kind of high asked me, 'Does everybody go religious on you?' A friend who walked her home after the workshop said that she was walking in the middle of the road singing at full volume. Perceptions also seems to change: colours are more clear and vibrant. There is love in the air!

Giving a hands-on treatment

During the workshop, you will be shown how to give a full Reiki treatment. The teacher demonstrates the hand positions and the students practice on each other. The treatment involves placing the hands in 16 positions on the patient's trunk and back in a set sequence. The legs and arms are not included unless the patient has a particular problem in that area or is extremely ungrounded. The Reiki will flow down to the limbs anyway. People often have tingling sensations there without any touch from the practitioner.

Length of time in each position

I used to be extremely careful to divide the one-hour treatment time between the 16 positions. But with experience, it became very natural to feel how much time I should spend in each position and I no longer had to think about it.

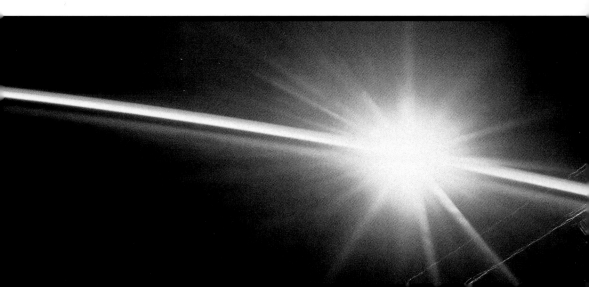

I found that my hands started moving by themselves. There is a strong connection between the heart and the hands. As the heart opens up through Reiki, the hands know what to do, and there is no need for interference from the mind.

Responding to the patient's needs

Sometimes the hands seem to get stuck in one position. There is a feeling of them being glued to the surface. This is a sign that the patient needs a lot of energy in this area. If your hand gets hot, there is too much activity in the area. You should stay in position until the heat has subsided. With cold it is the opposite – not enough energy, or old, stagnant energy. The place needs to be warmed.

If there is pain in the area you are treating, sometimes you will feel pain in your hands. The more serious the pain is, the higher up the arms you will feel the pain. As you continue to treat the patient, the pain will subside.

When you get a tingly sensation in your hands, it means that some kind of release is occurring. At times you can feel something like an electric shock going up your arm. That is also some sort of dramatic release. There can be a lot of variation in how you perceive things, but the general rule is that you should stay in an area as long as you sense that something is happening.

Hand positions for the front of the body

First position: forehead

Cover the patient's eyes with the palms on the forehead and the fingers pointing down towards the jaw.

Effects The heat from the hands relaxes muscle tension in and around the eyes, and, on a deeper level, the subtle energy penetrates the mind and calms thought processes. Sometimes you can feel thoughts like butterflies fluttering against your hands. The patient normally closes her eyes at this point and becomes deeply relaxed. The energy treats sinus problems and strengthens the pituitary gland. At the same time, the patient automatically pulls the energy to the area in the body where it is needed. This area usually gets very hot. When the heat subsides, move to the next position.

▲ First position: forehead

► Second position: temples

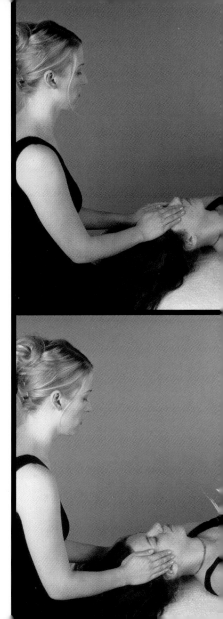

Second position: temples

Move the hands to the side so they cover the temples. The fingertips should touch the cheekbones. (You should not worry too much about the exact position: I have seen different Masters initiated by Takata all using slightly different positions.) As in all positions, the fingers are held loosely together to concentrate the energy.

Effects This position has the same effects as the first position and it is also good for side-headed headaches or migraines.

Third position: back of the head

Gently roll the head in your hands, so your hands are under the head, with the fingertips in the neck crease.

Effects As with all three head positions, this position is good for relieving headaches and for bringing heat downwards from the head. Having the head cradled in this manner can feel very safe for the patient. Reiki energy has a powerful effect on this area, which is where the head meets the neck and the spine. It helps to release muscular tension which otherwise disturbs the whole body mechanism. On a subtle level, all the main chakras are situated in line with the spine. I usually hold this position for quite some time.

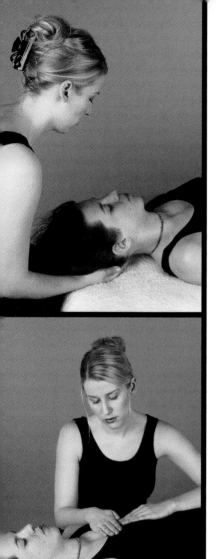

Fourth position: heart and lung

Put one hand below the collarbone and the other at right angles to it in the middle of the chest (so that the two hands form a 'T').

Effects On a physical level, this position is good for relieving asthma, bronchitis, and other respiratory complaints. Sometimes you can feel old, cold, stuck energy leaving like a wind over your hands. You may feel a muscular tightness that usually corresponds emotionally to a closed heart or emotional pain such as long-term grief or sadness. As this area opens up with Reiki, it is usually accompanied by an emotional release.

Wanja used to do this position from above the head of the patient. I find this too much of a stretch for my arms, so I do it from the side as I saw Mary McFadyon do, another of Takata's original Masters.

▲ Third position: back of the head

◀ Fourth position: heart and lung

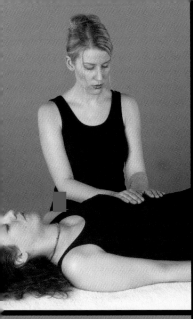

Fifth position: stomach and spleen

Place both hands on the lower ribs on the left side of the body covering the stomach and spleen.

Effects This position helps the digestion. Takata used to say that people treat their stomachs as garbage cans – they are not really conscious about what they eat. Sometimes she used to treat the digestive organs first – the stomach, spleen, and the liver – which shows the importance she placed on digestion.

Sixth position: liver

Move your hands to the opposite side of the body so that they cover the liver.

Effects There can be a sense of fullness and heat in this position, especially if the patient has a liver problem. On an emotional level, Reiki energy in this position can help to defuse anger. I once had a patient with quite a hot liver. I just said casually, 'Sometimes heat in the liver area corresponds to anger.' He quickly sat up, shouting, 'I AM NOT ANGRY!' The next day he

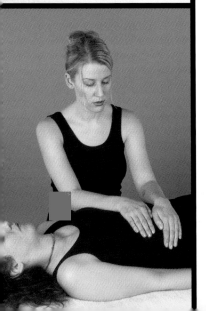

▲ Fifth position: stomach and spleen ◄ Sixth position: liver

told me that he had just read in an article that irritation was the same thing as anger. Maybe he was a little irritated, he confessed.

Seventh position: colon
Place your hands so they cover the transverse colon, roughly level with the belly button.
Effects This position helps with digestion and releasing waste matter. On an emotional level, the colon stands for letting go.

Eighth position: ovaries
The hands lie in a V-shape over the ovaries on women – one hand on each ovary. It usually gets very hot in this position.
Effects This placement is good for period pain and cramping. (Prostate problems are treated from the sacrum area.) It is also good for the bladder.

▼ Seventh position: colon   ▼ Eighth position: ovaries

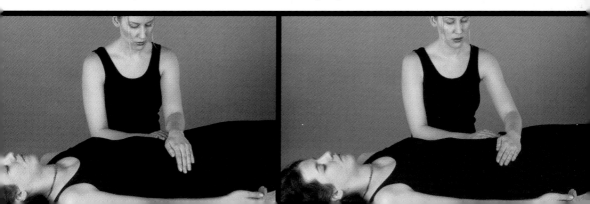

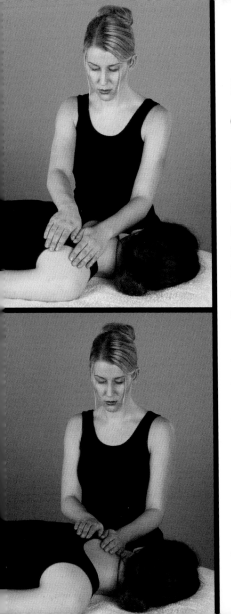

Hand positions for the back of the body

First position: right shoulder

Once the patient has turned over, locate the spine. Placing your hands in parallel, you are going to work on each side of the spine. I usually start with the right shoulder.
Effects This area of the body is where a lot of mental trauma is stored, which the Reiki energy releases.

Second position: left shoulder

Move your hands to the left shoulder.
Effects More physical problems are stored in this area. In addition, shoulders are often associated with responsibility and stress. We use a lot of expressions that mirror this fact, such as having 'a chip on your shoulder', and 'carrying the world on your shoulders'. Reiki helps to disperse tension from the area.

▲ First position: right shoulder   ◄ Second position: left shoulder

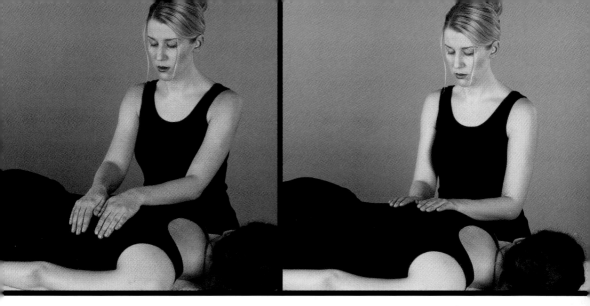

▲ Third position: right side of back   ▲ Fourth position: left side of back

Third position: right side of back

Place your hands together under the first position (the right shoulder).
Effects This releases postural muscle tension and tight backs. It also
affects the lungs and eases the breathing.

Fourth position: left side of back

Place your hands together under the left shoulder.
Effects Same as third position. Remember also that here you have the
back of the heart. All the back positions have a calming and soothing
effect. Working on the back feels like ironing out all the wrinkles.

Fifth position: kidneys

Place one hand on each of the kidneys, which are roughly located just above the waist.

Effects On an emotional level the kidneys are connected to fear. Often they can feel quite cold. You should stay in this position until they have warmed up a bit and feel balanced with one another.

Sixth position: lower back

Slide your hands down past the waist to cover the lumbar region, or the lower back.

Effects Reiki helps relieve the muscular tension that a lot of people suffer from in this area. Menstruating women often feel quite achy here too.

▼ Fifth position: kidneys

▼ Sixth position: lower back

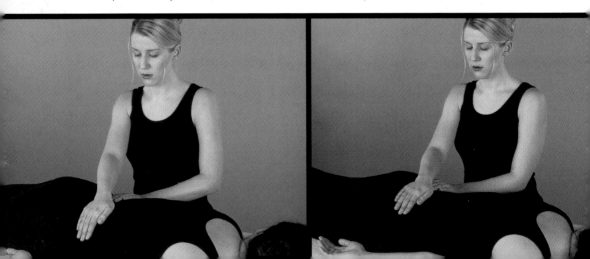

Seventh position: sacrum

Place your hands on the coccyx, or sacrum at the very bottom of the spine.
Effects This position is especially beneficial for men's prostate problems.

Final position: finishing the treatment

Put one hand at the top of the spine and keep the other on the sacrum. By this time, at the end of the treatment, the spine should feel quite open and you should feel a pulsation between your hands.
Effects End the treatment with an energy stroke to ground the patient and make her come back to her physical body. Using the index and middle finger of one hand with the other hand on top as a weight, run your fingers down each side of the spine in a downward stroke, usually three times.

Seventh position: sacrum ▲

Final position: finishing the treatment ▶

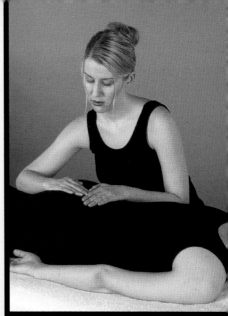

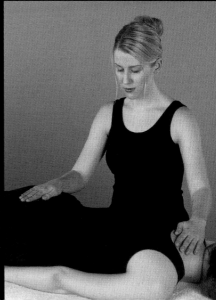

Patients' reactions

It can be interesting to listen to what people talk about when you have your hands on different parts of the body. One woman to whom I was giving Reiki responded emotionally as if I had pressed a button on each position in which I was putting my hands. On the heart area she started crying. When I moved my hands to her liver, she started talking about the anger that she felt towards her work colleagues. Her response when I had my hands on her shoulders was to talk about how stressed she was about everything she had to do – including writing a thesis. On the kidney area she got into her fear and worry about her son becoming a punk.

Intuitive empathy

While giving a Reiki treatment you are in a heightened intuitive space because of the link-up to higher energies while you are channelling. You might get flashes of intuitive knowledge about the patient and her condition or changes that would improve her health. This can come in the form of phrases in your head, seeing images, or just 'knowing'. Once I treated a patient going through a difficult phase in his marriage. I found that the phrase 'head and heart' kept repeating itself in my head and I realized that his problem was a total disconnection between his mind and his emotions.

Sometimes you might experience a strong physical and emotional reaction from the patient. I used to treat Diane for styes. As soon as I put my hands on her I was enveloped in a cloud of sadness and felt a deep pain in her heart. The sensation was so strong that I actually started to cry myself. It turned out that she was carrying around a great deal of pain and the fact that she could not cry when she was feeling emotional had resulted in the styes.

After the Reiki treatment, the styes disappeared and she felt much better inside. Every time I see her now she wants me to put my hands on her to feel if any pain is left in her heart.

This type of intuition has to be treated with delicacy – Reiki is not an encounter therapy, in which you tell people what is wrong with them and what they should do about it. It is much more valuable to give people space to come to their own conclusions. One method is to say 'I have a sense or a feeling of …' and to give the patient the option to reject or accept what you have to say. My teacher, Wanja, used to talk about somebody she knew whose case was similar to that of the patient. Unconsciously the patient would identify with the person in the story and would receive the message. I think this is a great non-confrontational method.

Self-treatment

It is while channelling Reiki that you are in direct contact with higher energies, and the purification of your body, mind, and emotions is accelerated. Takata always stressed the importance of starting the healing process with yourself.

In the beginning when I had just learned Reiki, I did not do much self-treatment. I could not feel the energy on myself in the same way as when I treated others. I also had trouble believing that anything could happen when I put my hands on myself. Only when I became more sensitive and I could feel the energy sizzling around my body when I treated myself, did I become convinced. Now I start every day with a self-treatment in bed for half an hour to an hour to link myself up to the energy source. It is rather like a meditation and it is also a bit like an internal scanning of the body to find out what is blocked and what needs a bit of tuning.

Giving yourself Reiki

The following are the classical self-treatment positions. It is not strictly necessary to follow the sequence or do all of the positions during the same treatment. You can also do the positions in any posture that you find comfortable – sitting, lying down or standing.

First position: forehead ▲

Second position: temples ▶

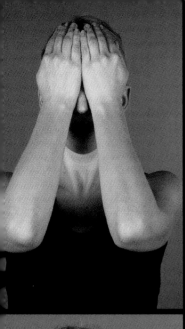

First position: forehead
Cover your eyes with your hands.

Second position: temples
With eyes closed, put your hands on your temples
in front of the ears.

Third position: back of the head
You can put your hands in any comfortable position on
the back of your head.

Third position: back of the head ▼

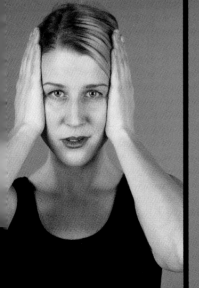

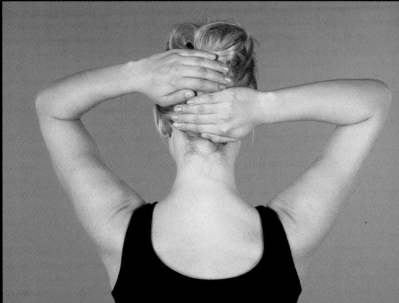

Fourth position: heart and lung

Place your hands in the middle of the chest.

Fifth position: stomach and spleen

Put the left hand on the left lower ribs covering the
stomach and spleen area and the right hand on
the right side of the lower ribs covering the liver.
The fingers should meet in the middle.

Sixth position: colon

Place your hands so they cover the transverse
colon, roughly level with the belly button.

Seventh position: ovaries and bladder

The hands lie in a V-shape over the ovaries on
women – one hand on each ovary.

Eighth position: kidneys

Place your hands above the waistline on your back.

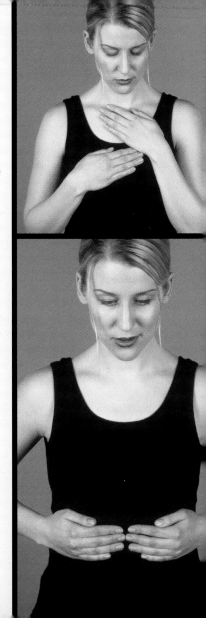

Fourth position: heart and lung ▲

From left to right: fifth position; stomach and spleen: sixth position; ▶
colon: seventh position; ovaries and bladder: eighth position; kidneys

You cannot comfortably treat the back, except the kidneys or lower back, which is best done in a sitting or standing position. Since the Reiki energy goes right through from the front, however, this is not a problem. I usually also suggest that people place their hands under the armpits to strengthen the immune system. In addition, it is a good idea for women to give Reiki to their breasts to cut the accumulation of stagnant energy and prevent the formation of lumps.

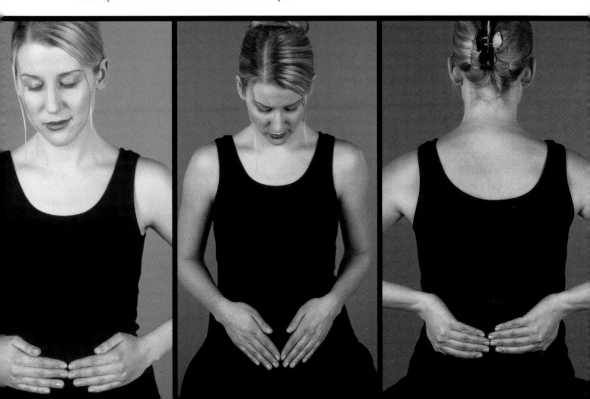

Of course, you can add any position you can comfortably reach! Again, it is important to understand that you do not have to go through the whole sequence of hand positions for self-treatment in one session: you can choose what is appropriate at any given time. Here are some suggestions for positions at different times of day:

After meals

After eating, place your hands on your stomach and liver to aid digestion. This is the fifth position described on page 46 and is also part of a qi gong exercise, a Chinese energy system for healing.

Going to sleep

When I go to sleep I always have my hands on the heart area in the middle of the chest, which is a very calming and nourishing position. (This is the fourth position described on page 46.)

Watching television

While watching television you can always have your hands somewhere on your body, since hands-on Reiki works automatically without any intention on your part. Put your hands anywhere where you have pain or feel tight.

Second Degree Reiki

What is second degree Reiki?

Second degree Reiki involves a further initiation, and it makes use of secret and sacred symbols. It deepens the inner personal transformation that started with the first degree Reiki.

In second degree Reiki you learn to heal at a distance, to work on a mental level to solve problems with people and situations, to 'clear' spaces, and to project wishes. You can also learn how to connect and communicate with animals and nature. An additional benefit of second degree Reiki is that it doubles the power of your hands-on healing. Takata used to say that first degree is like driving a car slowly at 30 miles an hour, whereas second degree is like stepping on the accelerator and driving at 80 miles an hour to get to your destination faster.

When should I learn second degree Reiki?

People who have learned first degree Reiki and feel enthusiastic about it usually decide to learn second degree. As a rule, it is good to wait a couple of months, so that the effects of the first degree Reiki initiation can settle. Some people wait years before they go on to the next step, and others are happy with just the first degree. It is a personal choice. If a person can handle the energy, it is possible to learn second degree Reiki straight after the first degree, and there are situations in which this is the most practical solution. Takata sometimes taught the second degree right after the first degree, for example in Canada when people had waited for her to come for a long time and had travelled long distances.

Why learn distant healing?

Often people want to learn distant healing because they have a family member or friend with some physical problem living in another city or even in another country, and they want to help. There was a woman in one of my second degree workshops, for example, who wanted to learn

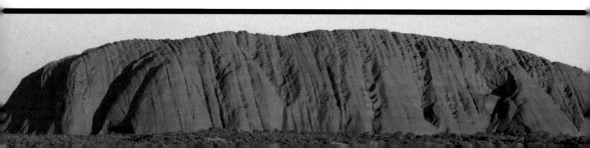

distant healing because her mother, who lived far away had a frozen shoulder. We were quite a big group sending the mother healing while practising. Straight afterwards we phoned the mother. She told us that she was having a shower at the exact time as we were sending her healing. Suddenly she noticed that she could stretch up the arm that was hardly movable before!

Not every case has such a dramatic outcome after just one distant Reiki treatment, but it is a great way to keep in contact with friends and family. I always start the day by sending some energy to my mother in Sweden. There is no limit to how often you can do a distant treatment. You can keep sending Reiki every day for serious problems.

First workshop day

The format of the second degree workshop is normally a couple of two-hour sessions held on consecutive days. We always start by sharing experiences people have had while practising first degree hands-on Reiki. It is really by using the Reiki on themselves, family members, and friends that people become convinced that Reiki works. I also answer any questions that come up about hands-on healing, and try to explain unusual experiences that people might have had. I want to be sure that there are no uncertainties left about first degree Reiki before we go to the next level.

The symbols

On the first day of the second degree workshop you will go through the symbols that are used for sending and projecting energy. These symbols should be given to you by a Reiki Master in combination with the second degree initiation. As they are secret and sacred, they must be treated with respect. The paper they are written on while practising should not be thrown away, but burned once the symbols have been learned by heart.

The symbols in themselves carry a certain energy even without the initiation. Once a man came back on the second day of a second degree workshop that I was running, rather puzzled. He said that when he came home after the first day he had a very strong emotional reaction. He was crying and trembling but he could not understand why, since in his words, 'we had not done anything.' I had to explain that his experiences came from drawing the symbols. The names of the symbols also carry energy. They function as mantras – holy sounds.

The power of the second degree lies in the combination of the drawing of the symbols, the sounds of their names and the initiation. You could say that the initiation activates the symbols. After the first day, the students take their copies of the symbols with them as homework to be learned by heart. Many students feel anxious that they will forget the symbols or not be able to remember them completely accurately. They just have to think back to when they learned the alphabet. In the beginning everybody carefully copied the teacher. Later, people developed all kinds of writing styles, but the letters still meant the same thing. It is the same thing with the symbols. The intention behind them is the important thing as long as they are recognizable.

It seems that Takata drew the symbols a little differently at times. I have compared the symbols that Takata gave my teacher Wanja with the way other Masters initiated by Takata draw them, and there are slight variations.

Second workshop day

On the second day of the workshop the students are initiated. There is only one initiation for the second degree, but it is a bit more elaborate than the initiations for the first degree.

Afterwards, we start the healing by working on each person's own issues. We sit in a circle and everybody in turn chooses something to work on with the group. Each person can choose between having a distant Reiki treatment, a distant mental Reiki working on some personal problematic situation or a wish. We usually finish the session by communicating with something uplifting such as trees, something else in nature or our guardian angels.

Since it can be difficult to believe that sending energy in this way really works, it is good to practise by sending it to the people in the group and then to compare notes. In this way you get immediate feedback. I remember being a bit of a 'doubting Thomas' myself when I first learned distant healing. To see if it worked, I put a friend with a headache in a corner of a room and started to send him some Reiki. While sending energy I kept asking, 'How does it feel now? How is your head?' Seeing his headache disappear little by little was the proof I needed. I think a bit of scepticism is quite healthy. The advantage of a group sending energy is that it is stronger and you can compare your sensations with other people's.

How to send Reiki

When you are sending distant or mental

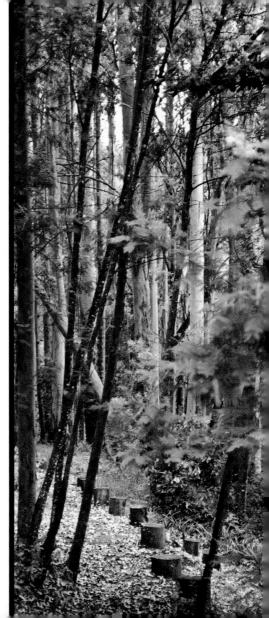

healing, you put your hands up in front of you so that you can sense the energy being pulled through you and out of your hands. The more energy the person or the situation needs, the more Reiki will be pulled through you. It can feel like heat, tingling or vibration in your hands. The second degree needs a little more focus than the first degree, so you usually keep your eyes closed while sending distant Reiki.

Since it is much more powerful than the hands-on healing, you only have to do up to 20 minutes instead of an hour. Sometimes not even that much time is needed, if there is no 'pull' in the hands and the energy feels quite settled.

In time, you will start picking up on the emotional states or physical pain of the person on whom you are working. Sometimes you can get intuitive information or see pictures in your mind. We try not to stop the flow of intuition by judging what is wrong or right, and also it is important not to treat this information as fact. It is essential, of course, to keep any information you pick up confidential.

As with hands-on Reiki, you are receiving a treatment at the same time as you are giving one, and as with hands-on healing, Reiki works regardless of how you feel. The things you pick up when you are working can have something to do with your own state of mind and personal 'stuff', but the more you practise, the more your intuition will grow, becoming clearer and clearer.

Questions people ask about distant healing

Does the exact distance matter?

When sending distant healing the actual distance is of no importance. The procedure for sending distant healing to a person in the same room or in a different country is exactly the same. Sometimes it is more convenient to do distant healing than hands-on, even if you are in the same place, for example if you are both in a car. Once I was in a taxi returning to New York from a meditation retreat. At the beginning of the two-hour journey the taxi driver complained about pains in his back and groin. I said I would try to do something about it. As we kept talking I was sending him distant Reiki. Just outside New York, I asked him how he was feeling, if he was still in pain. He was quite taken aback when he realized that his pain had disappeared. He was very pleased and said that if he had not worked for a company, he would have given me the ride for free.

Should the person give consent?

There is no need to ask permission from the person to whom you send distant healing. After all, you are just sending unconditional love. Who would refuse? There is also no need for the person receiving the Reiki to lie down or even to know the time when it is happening, though it can be interesting from a scientific point of view if they know that they are receiving Reiki.

Can you combine distant healing with hands-on?

In many cases it is practical to combine the first degree with the second degree Reiki. If, for example, it is difficult for a patient to come three or four days in a row for hands-on treatments, you can send a distant treatment instead.

What if someone does not want to be healed?

Once I was asked in a workshop to send healing to a woman who lived in the same house as one of my students and was suffering from cancer. She had refused conventional treatment and the other people in the house were terribly worried about her.

As we put up our hands, I felt something I have never felt before or since. It felt like hitting a brick wall; no energy went through it. Yet we knew that she needed it. Everybody in the group felt the same thing. The only thing I could think of was the fact that she had not asked for the healing herself. Maybe she wanted to go? So instead of sending Reiki to her, we started sending healing to all the other people in the house. Here it felt like a great need; it was as if the energy was being sucked out of our hands.

I think that sometimes, as healers, we want to heal everybody and everything and feel disappointed when this is not happening. It is important to have a detached attitude. We do what we can, but the result is not up to us. Maybe the physical tissues are too damaged, or maybe it is just time for the person to leave.

Mental healing

Mental healing is an aspect of distant Reiki. When sending mental healing you add a symbol that works as a key to open up your mind to another person's mind or to a situation. You can also use this symbol to communicate with animals and nature, to clear spaces or situations in the past or future and to project wishes. Because this kind of healing is much stronger than ordinary distant healing, you only need to send it for ten minutes for it to work.

When projecting specific energy to a person in this way, you need their permission. You also need to be very focused, because all your thoughts enter the other person. It is a reprogramming for mental problems, so you need to send positive affirmations or images. For example, if the person wants help for depression, you should send some positive emotion. If you decide to send joy, you have to visualize the person in a happy situation, repeat affirmations about the person being joyful, or create uplifting images from nature. If your mind wavers, you should stop.

Divine Order: another dimension of spiritual healing

If you want to send mental healing without visualizing the specific solution to the problem, you can just state the problem and add the phrase 'Divine Order' to the mental symbol. This type of healing is more like a prayer – you are sending the problem to the higher mind instead of manipulating the energy yourself. 'Divine Order' healing will only happen if it is part of the divine plan, and if it is good for the person. When you send mental healing in this way, you do not need to ask permission of the person.

I much prefer this way of working. This is also the way to work with problem situations and wishes. The only time I use the mental key without 'Divine Order' is when I want to communicate directly with animals, plants and other aspects of nature. I like to open the direct channels. I can send information but I can also stay open and receive at the same time.

How mental Reiki can help you

Mental Reiki may be used to make profound changes. It is a force for the good and it can literally change your life. Following are just some of the things it can help you to do:

Communicate with nature

A good way to replenish your energy is to use Reiki to connect to trees, rivers, mountains, oceans and even planets. Everything has its own energy pattern so you can tune into just what you need at the moment. Trees are especially good if you are feeling a bit 'ungrounded'. Connecting to trees, which have their roots in the ground and vertical trunk and crown in the sky, feels like having an Alexander lesson in which your spine lengthens and you open up to the world from a very supported position. To connect to oceans feels expanding and very relaxing, while making contact with volcanoes with all their inner activity is good for the digestion. Using Reiki to communicate with nature is a great way to make your own discoveries.

Realize your dreams

A great way to work with mental Reiki is to project your wishes. Because you use the

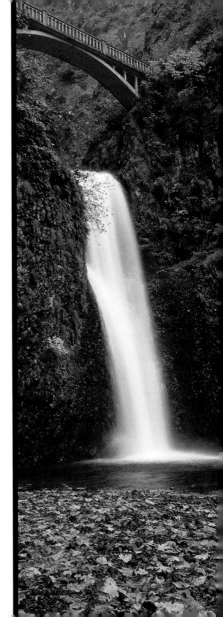

prefix 'Divine Order', you know that whatever you ask for will only happen if it is for your own good – if it is in the divine plan.

A woman to whom I was teaching second degree Reiki said she wanted to earn enough money to go to Peru and spend time with her shaman teacher, Juan. As we were formulating the wish, spontaneously I said, 'Me too!' I had for some time been interested in the shamanic way of healing. When we put our hands up I could feel an incredible energy coming into the room. I just said aloud, 'What is this?' The woman answered that it was her teacher, Juan. We sat with our hands up, pinned against the wall for about 45 minutes.

Some weeks later I happened to teach a few unusually big classes that left me with the exact amount of money I needed to go to Peru. I phoned a contact number in Brussels and found that there was only one place left in the group that was to work and travel with Juan. I was told to meet up with the group in a hotel in Lima on a certain date. I arrived at the hotel in the middle of the night. The next morning I saw a beautiful, very solid South American Indian, with long hair and a shining face, talking with some people. At first I thought it was a woman because of the softness of the gestures and posture. I was wrong – this was Juan.

I spent two incredible weeks with Juan, while he, in accordance with his tradition, tried to scare the living daylights out of me – we crossed wild rivers, crawled in underground tunnels, climbed mountains, and walked on the Inca pass where you almost die looking down into the deep abysses. I learned about Pacha Mamma – Mother Earth – and our connection to her. I had the most incredible experiences with energy and I must say that I have never seen such a beautiful country, situated high up in the clouds.

Open up the creative flow

One of my students in Paris, a painter, always does mental Reiki in order to connect herself to her inner creativity and intuition. I did the exact same thing before sitting down in front of my computer to write this book. For written tests and exams it is great to ask for clarity of mind and maybe also for a feeling of calm. People have asked me to send Reiki while they are delivering talks, and said they could feel the peacefulness of the energy descending on them.

Deal with the past

When dealing with energy there are no limits to time or space. You can use mental Reiki to go back in time and heal traumatic situations that occurred in childhood. I have worked in this way with a woman who was sexually abused. Some people who have experienced sexual abuse seem to be internally frozen in a state of fear. This is not just fear that comes from the initial abuse, but also fear of feeling in general, and sometimes an inability to access and express anger. Reiki can help to integrate and release these emotions. The woman told me that Reiki has helped to shift things for her. Of course, it is a slow process and she also does other things to help heal her early wounds.

Heal political situations

Sometimes local Reiki groups get together to send healing energy to bring peace to conflicts and political situations in different parts of the globe. During the Gulf War and other conflicts there was a lot of activities taking place on a subtle level, not just from Reiki groups, but from many different meditation and healing groups all around the world. A lot of healing energy was sent to that situation.

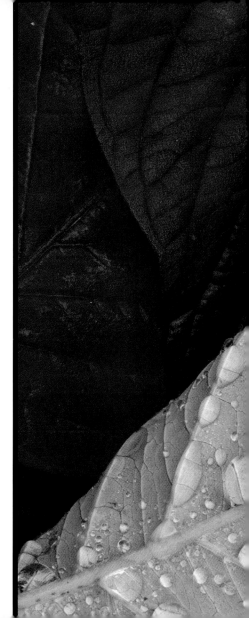

Living with Reiki

I think that Reiki should be a good habit that is completely integrated into your daily life, rather like brushing your teeth. In this section, I describe some inspiring events when Reiki has helped me and others, and brought a richness into my life.

Overcoming fear of the dentist

When I was little I developed a fear of dentists. I would dread my visits for months in advance. Even as I walked through the door, I would make him promise to give me an injection to kill the pain – just in case. As an adult, I had less fear since I chose a dentist who actually listened to me. But my fear had submerged to an unconscious level. When I had too many instruments in my mouth, I would involuntarily choke and spit them out. Apart from being uncomfortable, it was highly embarrassing and time-consuming.

   After I learned Reiki, I realized I could put one hand on my chest while my dentist was working and give myself Reiki to stop these gagging reflexes. Without Reiki I could never have gone through with having my amalgam fillings removed and replaced with a less toxic material. I spent hours in a relatively calm state with my excellent Swedish dentist, who ended up taking the Reiki initiations himself. I have also had the opportunity to assist a dentist in the US who specializes in root-canal treatment by giving Reiki to nervous patients with very good results.

Connecting with people through Reiki

In Sweden midsummer is celebrated all night long because of the light. One year, I offered Reiki to people suffering with hangovers after a heavy night drinking. I gave Reiki outside on the grass lawn since it was a glorious sunny day. Not only did the Reiki help the hangovers but I discussed very deep issues with many people. It was as if the Reiki cut through the social chit-chat to a level where things really mattered.

I especially remember a woman who was pregnant and was considering having an abortion because the nuclear accident at Chernobyl had just occurred and she was afraid that her baby might be damaged by radiation. Another person was contemplating a total change in his life and career. I cannot remember all the personal stories, but I do remember being moved and amazed at everything that was going on inside the people at the party.

I was giving Reiki practically continuously from morning to evening that day. I had my hands on somebody in the bus going to the beach.

On the way back to Stockholm I was with a woman who insisted on learning Reiki before I left for Devon, England, the next morning. Before she went home at midnight, she had her first initiations and practice. At six o'clock the next morning, she was back to receive her last initiations and she got her last-minute instructions as she helped me take my luggage to the bus for the boat to England. I was impressed with her dedication.

Helping an asthmatic

Being dyslexic and not very technically orientated, I never thought I could learn how to drive. However, a couple of years ago, I thought that I would take it up to see what would happen.

I talked about my problem to my acupuncturist, who recommended Jean as a driving instructor. One damp London day while sitting in the car, I felt a restriction in my chest and I found it difficult to breathe. I recognized the feeling from people I had treated for asthma, so I turned to my driving teacher and asked her if she had asthma. Jean looked quite startled and asked me how I knew. I then proceeded to explain about Reiki and offered to give her the initiations so we would both be able to breathe a bit better. I was also counting on Reiki having a calming effect during my driving lessons, which would benefit both of us. The effect of Reiki on Jean's asthmatic condition was truly amazing.

After the first day of the Reiki workshop she did not need to use the inhaler that she normally used twice a day.

Flying with Reiki

Returning by plane from Paris to London after a Reiki workshop, I sat down in my place. After a while I had the by now familiar sensation of a tightness around my chest and difficulty in breathing. I turned to the man in the seat next to me and asked him if he was suffering from asthma. He looked quite shocked and said, 'Are you a witch?' to which I answered: 'Certainly not!' I ended up treating him with distant Reiki all the way to Heathrow. He was quite intrigued and carried my luggage to the Underground.

To develop this kind of sensitivity is quite normal if you practice some kind of energy work for a long time, not just Reiki. It is just an extension of what you feel in yourself when you have your hands on somebody during a Reiki treatment. You can also tune into the state of somebody at a distance or in a picture if you choose to do so.

Accident in a Greyhound bus

I was travelling across the US in a Greyhound bus when a woman slipped on the floor. She fell so badly that she injured her back and could not move. The bus driver called for an ambulance to transport her to hospital. I had just recently learned Reiki and I was deliberating whether or not I should offer healing to the woman. Finally, I decided that I could offer it and let her decide. I was not thinking of curing her back but rather of treating her for the shock she suffered from the fall and lying immobile in the aisle of the bus. I went up to the woman and asked if I could give her some healing. She looked quite frightened and I could see what was going on in her mind – she could not cope with another strange thing happening to her. When she declined my offer, I asked if she wanted me to hold her hand instead. This time, her answer was yes. As I held her hand, I could feel her heart energy settle and I stayed with her until she was taken away to hospital in the ambulance. This incident taught me the importance of how you introduce Reiki. It is not necessary to offer complicated explanations about it being a several-thousand-year-old Japanese Buddhist system learned through initiations in India from a Swedish person. It is enough to touch and let the Reiki flow.

Motorbike accident in Nairobi

I was invited for dinner at the home of some friends in Nairobi. The host, Oscar, wanted to post a letter before eating and went off on his motorbike. His sister and I waited and I think an hour or so passed before somebody phoned to say that Oscar had been involved in a traffic accident. It took quite some time to locate the hospital to which he had been taken. He was lying in a ward waiting for a surgeon to come with a gaping wound on his forehead. One of his legs was also injured but I was more worried about his head injury. Oscar was still conscious and kept talking and moving non-stop as if not really aware of the seriousness of his injuries. As I started giving him Reiki on his heart area for shock, he felt very cold. Nobody stopped me giving him Reiki and I felt as though I was standing there for hours. Even while his forehead was being sewn together, I was allowed to do Reiki and talk and comfort him. Only when the surgeon came to operate on the leg did his sister and I have to leave.

The healing process was long, but throughout, Oscar did a lot of Reiki work himself on his leg. After a year he was fine. For me, it is not too important to know exactly what part Reiki played in the healing process. The value is more in the feeling that you can do something useful in situations like this. Often you get the feeling that you were meant to be there.

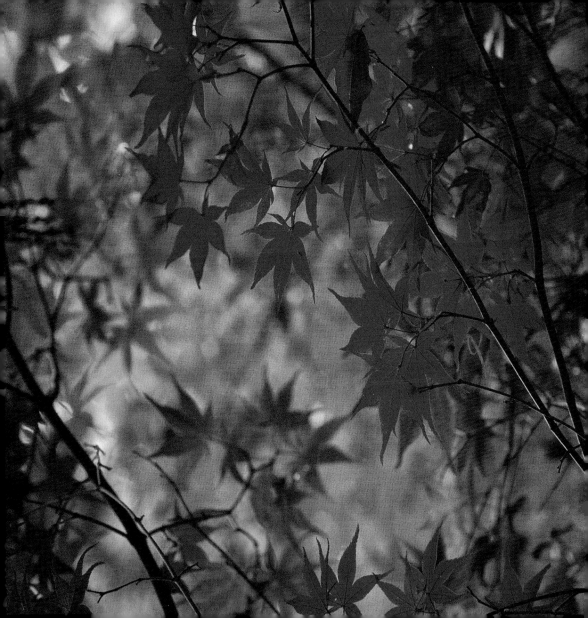

Reiki for Animals and Plants

I grew up in a home where everybody loved animals. Though we lived in a small town, we had a mini farm with cats, dogs, hens and rabbits in our garden. Even though my father was not a vet but a biology teacher, during winter people would bring starving, injured birds for him to care for at home. We all helped to feed and take care of them. Having this kind of background and love for animals made me look upon Reiki as a great gift. At last I had a tool for healing sick animals.

Different ways to treat animals

If an animal is tame, the easiest way to give to Reiki is hands-on healing. If possible, put your hands on the injured part of the animal. If this is not convenient, put the hands anywhere you can since, as with people, the Reiki energy goes where it is needed.

I find that animals enjoy Reiki. If there are animals like cats and dogs around while I am giving a Reiki class or a treatment, they usually place themselves on top of the patient. Even when the patient has left, they choose to lie down on the energy imprint left behind.

Animals, like children, tend to get very hot during a Reiki session, so the treatment tends to be shorter than an hour. If the heat of the Reiki makes an animal restless, you can just caress it. If you lift your hands when stroking it makes the treatment less intense and the animal is

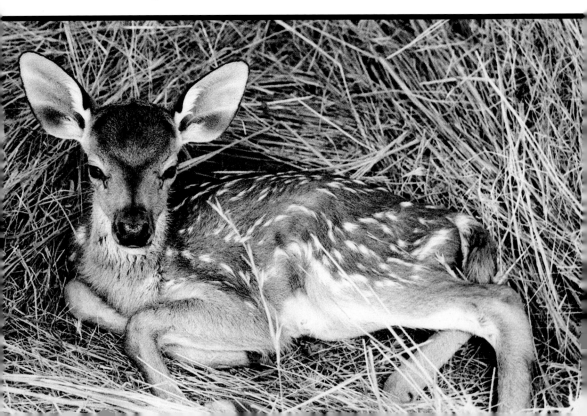

used to and understands your behaviour. The Reiki will come through anyway.

As water conducts energy, it facilitates the flow of Reiki. Putting our hands in the animals' drinking water to energize it was a practice that my teacher Wanja and I used while healing deer in an ashram in India. Another way to use water to intensify the treatment is to rinse a towel in water and put it on the animal with your hands over it while giving Reiki. This is especially practical for big animals such as cows or horses as it is difficult to put your hands all over their bodies.

For wild animals and when the animal is not present, distant Reiki is extremely convenient. Mental Reiki is great for communication and solving behavioural problems in animals.

Healing deer

In India I was in charge of a herd of deer for six years. While taking care of them, I learned Reiki. During mating season, there was a lot of fighting between the male deer. I especially remember a deer that had an antler poked into its eye.

The eye was so swollen that it looked as if it was going to pop out of its socket. I kept feeding him carrots while putting my hand over his injured eye. After a couple of days the eye sunk into the socket with the cornea looking like a folded clear tape. The eye looked milky and opaque and seemed to have no sight. Meanwhile, a pocket of pus, big as a fist, was forming underneath the eye. I kept giving Reiki since I did not want the other eye to get infected too, and leave him blind in both eyes. I certainly had to learn not to be squeamish, as the pus started to pour out underneath the eye. After a week the swelling had reduced, the eye came back to its normal position, the cornea stretched out again, and the colour of the eye went back to normal. I realized that the deer could see with it again.

Reiki for trees and plants

In the same way that animals like Reiki, so do plants. Reiki does not just go in a linear way from practitioner to patient. When Reiki is practised, an energy field is created. A clairvoyant who watched

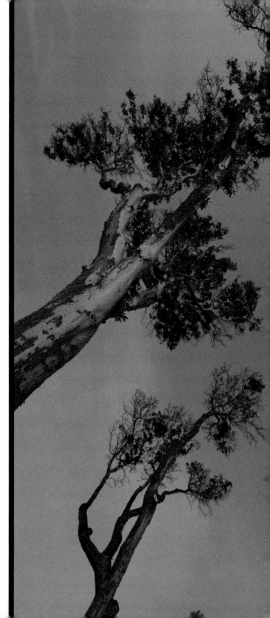

me giving a Reiki session saw an orange cloud of energy coming out of my body as I started the session. After the Reiki treatment it took about five minutes for the cloud to vanish. This field of energy, or life force, makes plants flourish. You can always tell what is going on in a place by looking at the state of the plants.

The first time I did healing on plants was in the ashram in India. I was asked by one of the gardeners to give some healing to a few bushes that had been replanted. I thought he just wanted to be nice to me, knowing that I had just learned this new 'thing' – Reiki. As I put my hands on the stem of one of the bushes I did not expect anything particular but I was in for a surprise.

I could actually feel the trembling and shock inside the bush. I was feeling the reality of the expression that a plant goes into shock when replanted.

Later I did a lot of distant healing on trees that had been replanted and they felt the same, only stronger.

Working on plants, you can either cup your hands around them or touch their stems. You can also energize the water that you use for watering with Reiki. Holding seeds for a while in the hands before planting is another way of giving Reiki energy. One of my students used to give her whole garden distant Reiki. It is just a question of being creative. Anything is possible!

Healing horses

The first horse owner I taught Reiki to was a woman in New Mexico with 25 polo horses. She learned both first and second degree Reiki so she could care for the horses herself they got any injuries while she was transporting them from New Mexico to California. She had no problems understanding the concept of mental and distant healing, since she felt that she already had a very strong telepathic connection with her horses.

Danny, a riding school teacher and Alexander teacher, was so impressed with the Reiki healing that a friend of mine did on one of his horses that he wanted to learn it himself. He later invited me to give a class to other people at his riding school. I always love to teach Reiki to people who love animals since animals have played such an important part in my life.

The kinds of problems Danny thinks Reiki has helped the horses with are: discomfort and pain, swellings, muscular strains, sprains and stress. He has also had success treating colds and infections such as glandular swellings behind the ears. Fadie, a dog living at the riding school, has become a bit of a Reiki addict. He will get close to Danny and demand Reiki by putting forward the body part he wants to be treated.

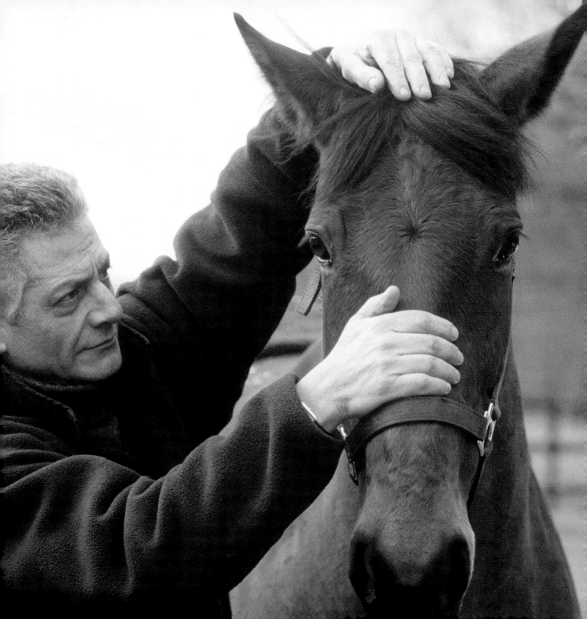

Combining Reiki with Other Therapies

Reiki can be combined with any other healing method; nothing is contraindicated. Reiki just means life force – it is totally natural. Whatever healing or body work you do will only be enhanced by Reiki.

Once you are initiated, you cannot actually turn off the Reiki. It is part of your energy system. I will give examples of how Reiki can add an extra dimension to other alternative healing and educational systems of which I have personal experience. Reiki can also be very successfully combined with orthodox medicine.

Reiki and massage

Having learned Reiki, I became curious about other complementary therapies and started a three-month course of Swedish massage. During the course I taught Reiki to many of my fellow students. While giving massage there was a marked difference in the heat of the hands of the students who had Reiki and those who did not. The clients would say, 'Oh, you have nice warm hands!' Of course, massage from someone initiated in Reiki has the added effect of the healing energy penetrating on a deeper level at the same time as the muscle tension is released. When working at a Swedish health farm, I gave a very perceptive little old lady a massage. After the massage, she asked me, 'What was that other thing coming out of your fingers?'

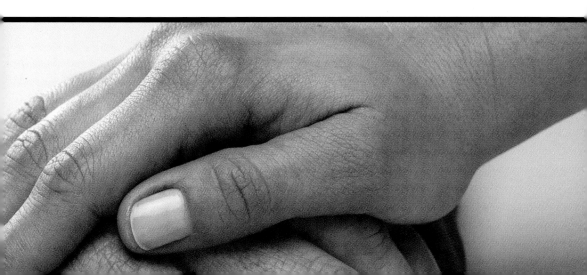

The only difference between a pure Reiki session and a massage from someone trained in Reiki is that the former is somewhat stronger since the hands are in contact with the body the whole time.

A benefit if you are trained in Reiki and practise massage or other types of body work is that the energy protects you from picking up negative vibes from your clients. Also because the Reiki is flowing all the time while you have body contact, you will get less tired.

Reiki and the Alexander Technique

The Alexander Technique is a system of re-education in which we are taught to become conscious of our postural habits and how we use ourselves in daily activities. Along with verbal instructions, the Alexander teacher uses his hands to guide the pupil in her movements to bring about better coordination.

Having trained in the Alexander Technique, I used to treat people with bad back problems. I used Reiki to help ease tension and release backs that had gone into spasm. Even when bones had gone out of their proper alignment, they would return once the muscles were released. Normally, patients would only need three Reiki sessions on consecutive days. I once treated an elderly Australian woman whose whole back had seized up and was made worse after somebody had tried to treat her with massage. She could not move at all. When somebody has had the wrong treatment there is, understandably, a lot of fear involved. Because of the non-invasive, 'non-doing' character of Reiki, it was perfect for this woman. It took about a month of regular Reiki treatments to relieve the tension in her back and for her to regain mobility. She ended up learning Reiki herself, as do most people who have experienced amazing healings.

Having the Reiki initiations would not change the way an Alexander teacher teaches. In my experience it would only affect the quality of the touch. It is a very subtle difference. I also feel that Reiki helps open up the intuition and sensitivity that is important in Alexander work. It is just part of you if you have the Reiki initiations – a bonus.

Qigong and Reiki

Qigong, which consists of sets of special exercises and meditations, is part of the traditional Chinese way of strengthening health, relieving illness, prolonging life, improving mental health, and achieving high levels of self-realization. Qi means energy or life force, and *gong* means cultivate or accumulate.

I think that Reiki and Qigong have a lot in common. Both are ancient oriental systems taught through initiation or transmission from a teacher and are based in similar traditions. Both are spiritual practices in which the main purpose is healing – in the fullest sense of the word.

The main difference is the movement in the Qigong practice, which complements Reiki practice, in which you sit still for hours. Because people who are initiated into Reiki are used to sensing energy, it is very easy to teach them qigong.

Acupuncture and Reiki

Acupuncture, like Qigong, is part of Traditional Chinese Medicine. Needles are inserted to manipulate or balance vital energy, which flows in channels or meridians around the body.

I find acupuncture a quick remedy for acute and very specific complaints. It also combines well with Reiki. When I started having acupuncture, I never thought about the fact that you, as a patient, would get the acupuncturist's energy through the needles. Now, with more experience, I think that this is obvious. So not only can an acupuncturist with Reiki give hands-on healing to the patient while the needles are in position, but the energy going into the needles will be purer and stronger.

I once gave Reiki to two patients who were HIV-positive. At the same time, they were being treated with acupuncture by another practitioner to strengthen their immune systems. When I put my hands on their feet, I had the most curious feeling. It was like plugging my hands into an energy field that was already in existence. I also felt the emotional turmoil these men were going through, but soon could sense the soothing effect of the Reiki taking place. It felt like two healing channels at work at the same time.

Reiki and other complementary therapies

Bach Flower Remedies are infusions of flowers or plants in homeopathic dilutions that are given to help negative emotional states. When I first started treating people who had emotional problems, I used to prescribe Bach Remedy drops to be taken between treatments to speed up the healing. It is easy to prescribe the appropriate remedies since you get to know a person's particular problem very well while treating them.

I know a Reiki practitioner who sends many of her patients to get homeopathic remedies from another practitioner and finds that Reiki and homeopathy make an excellent combination. The only problem when doing combined treatment is being able to tell which treatment did what, if that is important to you.

A way to increase the efficacy of a homeopathic, herbal, or other remedy is for a Reiki practitioner to hold the bottle or herbs in their hands so that Reiki energy is absorbed into the remedy. Some people use this technique even for orthodox drugs to minimize any bad side effects. Crystals can also be empowered by Reiki, by holding them in your hands or by using mental programming on them.

Reiki with orthodox medicine

It is important when practising complementary medicine not to prevent people from taking orthodox medicine. On no account should you tell them to stop conventional drug treatment. This is a matter between them and their doctors. Reiki sometimes has miraculous results, but healing is not something that you as a practitioner can promise your patient – it is not in your hands.

If a person wants to use only complementary methods to help the healing process, it is his or her personal choice. Apart from Reiki, there are many other ways to improve health, for example making changes to diet and lifestyle, looking at the spiritual dimension of life and starting to practise systems such as yoga or Qigong.

Also, a combination of complementary therapies might be helpful.

There is no contraindication to using Reiki alongside conventional medicine – in fact it can greatly help those undergoing conventional treatment. Jan, for example, a woman in her early fifties, had cervical cancer. As surgery was not an option, a series of 30 sessions of radiotherapy was planned. Halfway through her treatment she started having Reiki, but by this time was feeling very unwell. Because of Jan's poor condition, Migi, her practitioner, suggested to Jan that she should take the Reiki initiations so that she could treat herself every day. A few weeks later Jan was initiated by me into first degree Reiki. Even though Jan gave herself Reiki every day, she continued her Reiki sessions with Migi once a month. Slowly during the summer, Jan started to regain her strength and the burns she had suffered as a side effect of the cancer treatment began to heal.

Jan believes her recovery from the damaging effects of radiotherapy was accelerated through Reiki treatments. She thinks that Reiki minimized some of the possible damage to her bowel and her bladder, and that it helped to shrink the tumour and heal the effects of the radiotherapy. The latest scan shows no sign of the tumour. Another benefit of the Reiki is that Jan is no longer experiencing headaches, which had been a long-term problem. Now Jan looks great!

The Five Reiki Spiritual Principles

Here are Dr Usui's five spiritual principles of Reiki, which are guidelines on how to live. They might seem simple, but they are not always so easy to follow. Use them as a focus for meditation.

Just for today do not anger

This does not mean that we should repress anger. It means that we should be conscious of our feelings and try to communicate them in a constructive way – not dump our anger on people who have nothing to do with it. Whenever there is a mismatch between the intensity of the feelings and the event that has taken place, we know there are a lot of unconscious feelings bubbling to the surface. The more we connect to the real love inside, the faster we can let go of anger and other negative emotions. There is nothing wrong with feelings. Emotion is just energy that keeps moving. It is when it gets stuck that we become ill.

Just for today do not worry

Worrying does not help any issue or situation. It only creates tension and stress. If we truly realize this, we can drop the worrying like a bad habit. Just for today, we can try to experience the support that is all around us. If we worry a lot, it shows our disconnectedness from the divine; there is a lack of trust. Use whatever means you know to connect again: prayer, meditation, and Reiki.

Honour your teachers, parents and elders

We learn from our parents and teachers. When we take their knowledge inside us, it becomes part of us. So to honour parents and teachers is to honour ourselves.

  My parents always supported me, even if sometimes they did not understand what I was doing. I will always be grateful for that. Even if you do not agree with everything your parents did, they in their turn were victims of their parents. So you have to look upon them with understanding and compassion. To keep blaming is to be locked into a reactive pattern.

Thinking of my teachers, I feel enormous gratitude. There is no way that I can pay them back for their precious gifts. I can only try to follow their teachings.

Earn your living honestly

We must live our lives in a way that keeps us true to ourselves. The moral way in which we conduct our lives will, in the widest sense, reflect on our health. Honesty is not just about keeping to the facts. It is about honouring our deepest feelings and beliefs and being aligned to the divine power inside.

Show gratitude to all living things

In Reiki we always end a treatment by saying, 'Thank you, thank you, thank you!' This acknowledges the work of the spiritual energy. We are only its channels. People, animals, plants – we are all interconnected by Reiki energy. When we truly realize this, we start living with compassion and love, entering our true state of being.

Useful Addresses and Websites

The Reiki Association

2 Manor Cottages
Stockley Hill
Peterchurch
Hereford HR2 0SF
www.reikiassociation.org.uk

The Reiki Alliance

US Office:

The Reiki Alliance
PO Box 41
Cataldo, Idaho 83810—1041
USA
Tel: 1 208 682 3535
Fax: 1 208 682 4848
E-mail: ReikiAlliance@compuserve.com
www.reikialliance.org.uk

European Office:

Stichting The Reiki Alliance – Europe Office
PO Box 75523
1070 AM Amsterdam
Netherlands
Phone: + 31(0) 294 290022
Fax: + 31(0) 294 290931
E-mail: 100125.466@compuserve.com

Reiki Outreach International

PO Box 609
Fair Oaks
CA 955628
USA
Tel: + 1 916 863 1500

Further Reading

Kajsa Krishni Boräng **Principles of Reiki** Thorsons, 1997

Fran Brown **Living Reiki Takata's Teachings** Life Rhythm, 1992

Helen J. Haberly **Reiki: Hawayo Takata's Story** Archedigm, 1990

Marie Hall **Practical Reiki** Thorsons, 1997

Tanmaya Honervogt **Reiki: Healing and Harmony Through the Hands**

Gaia Books Ltd, 1998

Wanja Twan **In the Light of a Distant Star** Morning Star Productions,

British Columbia, Canada 1995. Can be ordered from Box 407, Kaslo

BC, Canada Vogimo